Paul Lindell, through his own experience of suffering, has shown us how to face the mystery of pain. The biblical insights and applications will help his fellow sufferers to face pain realistically and honestly. To better understand the exigencies of life on this planet is to better comprehend God's purpose for our lives. After reading this superb book pain is less a mystery for me than before, and more an instrument of God's grace.

Conrad Thompson

The *Mystery of Pain* by Paul J. Lindell moves into an area of life where we meet many unanswered questions. His very realistic searching of the Scriptures for answers, and his analyzing them very frankly, makes this a must for everyone who knows that sooner or later pain may be his lot in life.

W. E. Klawitter

A truly brilliant discourse on the problem and purpose of suffering—brilliant in the light of divine revelation and Spirit-filled theological insights given to God's servant. From his deep valley of infirmity and pain, Paul Lindell shares with us his view of the Son of Righteousness who comes with the reassuring word, "My grace is sufficient for you."

William E. Berg

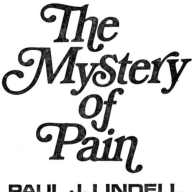

The Mystery of Pain

PAUL J. LINDELL

AUGSBURG PUBLISHING HOUSE
Minneapolis, Minnesota

THE MYSTERY OF PAIN

Copyright © 1974 Augsburg Publishing House

Library of Congress Catalog Card No. 74-77676

International Standard Book No. 0-8066-1424-2

Scripture quotations are from the Revised Standard Version of the Bible, copyright 1946, 1952, and 1971 by the Division of Christian Education of the National Council of Churches and are used by permission.

MANUFACTURED IN THE UNITED STATES OF AMERICA

Contents

Preface

My generation, by and large, is inquisitive and unafraid of the world and of living in this world the way it is. It is true that the problems of life do put a scare into some people and they drift off to the sidelines. But for most of us these problems are simply the stuff we have to work with to make life on this planet what we want it to be.

This makes us problem conscious. Our approach to almost anything and everything, large or small, is the problem-solving approach. We go into education or science, politics or management, human relations or industry, and even into art and religion as problem areas. We sort out the problems that exist. We then analyze them thoroughly. After theorizing and experimenting we pounce on whatever workable solutions we find.

My generation is asking *does* questions. What does it do? Why does it go wrong? How do we fix it? This persistent curiosity is being constantly rewarded with new discoveries, new products, and new conquests in the use of time and space.

But there are some crucial and baffling problems that are way beyond us. They seem to arise out on the dark edges of our existence, at the point of our entry and at the point of our departure.

At the one frontier (of birth) we are about to swarm and overstuff the world with people. At the other frontier (of death) we have triggered a monstrous power that can wipe out the human race with a few loud bangs.

Meanwhile, between our exits and our entrances, we live in encircling gloom, an envelope of pain and distress. Afflictions and illness, disorder and conflict are ever with us. Somehow things are not what they ought to be. There is a rot and decay in everything. There are limitations that cannot be extended even for what is most noble and beautiful. There are evil powers that prowl the earth untamed.

Not all of our *does* questions fit here. These conditions are different in kind as well as in degree from every other problem with which we have to deal. We must here ask another type of question. Now we will have to ask *is* questions. What is the meaning of life? Why are we here? Who is in control of the world and the universe? Where is our destiny? Are we responsible? What shall we do to be saved?

But I must be personal about this, for letters come to me from fellow missionaries in other parts of the world who are baffled and hurt. Illness, pain, and loss force colleagues to leave their posts and those that remain are overburdened. One writes about this with a sob of anguish in her heart. In distress she asks why this happens. Why cannot God's servants be kept from "the pestilence that stalks in darkness, and the destruction that wastes at noonday?" Or when it comes, why cannot we find protection? Why cannot we obtain healing and deliverance, health and strength? Is God not able and willing to give this? Is it because we are weak in faith? Or is it because we do not know how to work miracles?

I must also be personal about this for another reason. Some time ago a doctor firmly closed the door of his office and then said to me, "I'll give it to you straight. You have cancer." Suddenly in a new way I was face to face with the ultimate frontier. The pains, ills, distresses, and sorrows that plague men and women everywhere now had a firm hold on me. How shall I meet this?

1

The Mystery of Pain

There is a mystery about pain, suffering, illness, sorrow, and death. If all of this were merely a problem, philosophy or theology could look for an answer. Or, if pain were no more than a maladjustment of some kind, the medical people, or the science people could find ways to cure it. But pain, however it comes, is an event. And that is how the Bible meets it. It does not give us some neat, logical answer to the puzzle of pain, for there is none. It is plainly a mystery. What makes it so?

Pain Is Real

Pain, in the widest sense, is not imaginary. It is not some bad dream that comes on a hot summer night. It is real, actual, not academic. It happens. It hits a person and it may hit suddenly, blindly, even madly. It is a shock and it hurts acutely.

Pain comes from all directions. It may come from natural disasters, as it did to Job. Or it may come from historical causes, as it did to Israel at the destruction of Jerusalem and the captivity and exile into Babylon. In any case it is real. It is tragic. It makes one silent, sober, numb. This is because we sense, when we are smitten with pain, that it is a mystery.

Pain Is Constitutional

It is in the nature of men to suffer. "Man is born to trouble as the sparks fly upward" (Job 5:7—from the speech of Eliphaz the Temanite). And now the questions come thronging. Is this really so? How can it be? Why must this be so? What about undeserved pain? What has gone wrong? Surely this is not the way things should be. How can we fix things up to make them work out as they should?

The simple truth is, we cannot escape pain. It does not come in the same form or in the same measure to all people alike, but it does come to all. It goes right down into the roots of our human nature and life. We can feel it in our bones. And that is part of the awesome mystery.

The Question of Responsibility

When pain comes we feel that we are somehow responsible, even though we did not originate it or do something to bring it on.

This idea is vaguely felt in the pagan world. Hindus and Buddhists have built their whole outlook on life around this feeling. Science, too, following the cause and effect pattern, looks for reasons for pain and suffering and feels responsible to somehow find and make a cure for people.

"Who sinned," asked the disciples, "this man or his parents, that he should be born blind?" Somebody must certainly be responsible for causing this pitiful condition!

Deuteronomy teaches and preaches this idea as a true doctrine. And it was on this assumption that the comforting friends insisted that Job must be covering up some sins, for surely the evils that were on him were a just punishment for wrongs done. He must be responsible!

On a higher level perhaps, some people say that we do not have more divine healing because we are too weak in faith, too carnal in spirit, too unfit to receive healing from God for those who are sick among us. Thus we are responsible for the continuance of pain. And all of this also adds to the puzzling mystery of pain.

What the New Testament Says

The New Testament does not teach that God sends pain, yet it is open about saying that God allows it to come.

- Simon, Simon, behold Satan demanded to have you, that he might sift you like wheat, but I have prayed for you that your faith might not fail (Luke 22:31-32). *God allowed the satanic sifting and trial.*

• We know that we are of God, and the whole world is in the power of the evil one (1 John 5:19). *God allows this!*

• About that time Herod the king laid violent hands upon some who belonged to the church. He killed James, the brother of John, with the sword (Acts 12:1-2). *And God didn't stop him!*

Over and over again, as with John the Baptizer, good and holy people have been put to death at the hands of evil men, or they have withered away from inner tumors, or they have starved in times of disaster while God seemingly stood by and did absolutely nothing to deliver them.

Some have suffered torture, illness, famine, exposure, loneliness, temptation, or mental disorders, and there has been no deliverance. Must I not then say that somehow God seemingly allows this to happen, just as he allowed the very worst of evils to fall upon his own beloved Son? His enemies watched as the soldiers nailed him and raised him up on the cross. They stripped him naked and mocked and derided him, saying, "He trusts in God. Let God deliver him now, if he desires him; for he has said, 'I am the Son of God.'" But no deliverance came—not from God in heaven, nor from his friends and followers. Then in an agony of despair Jesus cried, "My God, My God, why hast thou forsaken me?" And this deepens the mystery of pain.

The Problem of Deliverance

The power and willingness of Jesus to deliver from pain is surely unlimited. And he has promised this power to be used by his followers too. We know this. But we stand helpless in the midst of a stricken world that bleeds, and suffers, and weeps for all the pains that hurt so much. Only now and then do we see someone who is able to throw off pain and go home well and whole. Some stand up and shed their pains like old garments while others are wrapped up in the same pains as in a shroud and are carried off to their graves. No amount of medicine, surgery, prayer, anointing with oil, laying on of hands, or fasting and prayer has been able to bring healing to some of those we would most like to see healed. Therefore we have hospitals and institutes and homes for vast numbers of people whose pains are considered to be beyond repair. Why is this? Why is this? Why is the gap between God's healing power and our need for healing and deliverance so wide and unbridgeable? And so the mystery stubbornly remains.

Satan and Demonic Powers

That Satan and demonic powers deal in pain is openly declared in the Scripture. Some people are bound, afflicted, tempted, deceived, sifted, oppressed, made to be sick, and are even killed by demonic attacks. Jesus cast out spirits that sometimes crippled, weakened, or crazed people. Satan is a foe we cannot see and cannot fight in any ordinary way. He is crafty, evil, murderous, and goes about seeking someone to devour.

We know that even when demons do not possess people they can stir up storms of fear, anxiety, resentment, yearning, or despair that may bring ulcers, heart attacks, kidney trouble, or headaches.

On the other hand, the converse also seems to be true. Where demons have been worshiped as gods, or where experienced witches know of ways to enlist the help of powers in this unseen world of spirits, people obtain healing and restoration from all kinds of maladies. It is possible to bring benefits on crops and animals as well. Some men by careful discipline and with the help of spirits can overcome many limitations. They can communicate by thought transference with others at great distances. They can speed, almost weightless, over the ground for days without fatigue. They can insulate themselves from the deep-freeze of winter blasts, as well as the boiling heat of summer suns. They can walk unharmed amid the perils of fire, water, plague, or foe.

Added to this is the Bible's disclosure that the devil is in a way a servant of God. We do not know how or why this mighty foe should be allowed to have such a free hand in the world, but we are assured that even his worst attacks can be turned by God into blessings. Of course the supreme example of this is the cross where Satan entered into Judas who then carried out the dastardly plot to kill Jesus. There on Calvary Satan did his worst. But Jesus took his worst and out of it God wrung the redemption of the world.

Yet knowing all of this does not relieve us of our present pains. It only adds complexity to the mystery

2

Three Responses to Pain

How do people meet pain when they *do not* meet it at the cross of Jesus?

The Attempt to Sidestep Pain

There are many helps in this old mixed-up world to keep people from facing up to pain. Some try to sidestep it.

- For physical pain there are drugs, anesthesia, and acupuncture.

- For the terrors of war some can say, "Oh well, I'm not eligible for the draft" or "I'm a conscientious objector."

- For disaster there are those who say, "Let the government or the Red Cross take care of it."

- For death, accident, or other troubles that come to people, the neighbors may just look the other way and think it prudent not to become involved (as in the story of the Good Samaritan).

Buddhism offers a way of enlightenment to rid the mind and soul of pain. Just look at the image of Buddha, set up by the millions all over Asia. He is the Blessed One. His face is like a mask—tired, drained, impassive, cynical. The eyes look out on the pains of life unseeing, unmoved, unresponsive. This is the symbol for the world's greatest way to deliberately and systematically evade pain.

Christian Science sidesteps pain by calling it an "error of mortal mind." But how can this be a sensible and honest way to look at the pains of millions who are crippled in body by accidents and war, or the millions who are mentally broken and helpless, or the millions who are stunted by poverty?

Sidestepping pain, by whatever method, never really succeeds. Though it may seem to work for a time in a man's thinking, it fails to heal anything at the center of life. Men may try to lock the door against misery and keep it out, but it has a way of working in through the cracks, or of waiting outside until one day it can burst in when the door is opened.

Repression or denial of pain brings other ills. If you plaster down a boil the infection spreads beneath the skin and breaks out in other places. The sidestepper lives in an unreal world. His fears become fantasy. At length he may become brutish and there will be no truth left in him.

Hinduism has for ages been a way of sidestepping pain by teaching that all ills in this life come from wrongs committed in a previous life. Pain is simply a matter of cause and effect. For this reason men looked at each other without sympathy, for even the deepest distress was but reaping what had earlier been sown. Thus there is no help for it.

But modern India is finding this unworkable in the present day and is tearing out this age-long foundation stone in the Hindu structure. With determined courage India is now resolved to get rid of poverty, ignorance, pain, and inequality. And this India is doing on the altogether new and tacit assumption that these ills are not inevitable and must no longer be uncritically accepted and suffered. This is a brave idea but it runs into a dead end. The ills remain.

The Response of Radical Endurance

The Stoics of long ago left a lasting mark in history by their radical endurance of suffering. Deliberately, methodically, thoughtfully, and quietly they strangled all questions about pain and just took on the chin whatever came.

Stoics of a sort live all around us. Some are very thoughtful, logical, and sophisticated in their thinking. They root their attitudes in the icy reasoning and tests of objective science and then look with apathy on whatever happens.

But the general run of hometown Stoics have a watered-down kind of stoicism and express their attitudes in a common lingo we all know.

- Well, that's how thing go. Better like it or lump it.

- That's how the cookie crumbles, or that's how the ball bounces.

- What will be will be (the theme of a popular song a while back).

- What's the matter, Bud? Can't you take it?

- What can't be cured will have to be endured

- Buck up, old kid, play the man. You got what it takes!

But this kind of stuff is shallow and thin.

It won't stand up. It has little or no room for pity, grief, joy, or hope. Its realism is only pretended, for it does not look at life honestly, steadily, or as a whole. There is no open window to heaven and it looks for no tomorrow. Such a way of meeting the pains of life is hopeless, because it is born dead.

The Response of Rebellion

A third way of responding to pain is in outright rebellion. This can take low forms, as when a man turns in bitterness away from God and his Word and his church when some tragedy comes. A missionary dentist in China lost his son in a drowning accident. He questioned the faithfulness of God. This led to complaint and murmuring and finally issued in bitter revolt. He left the light of walking with God and lost himself in the gloom of the perishing world around.

But rebellion can also take high forms, as when Gandhi devoted his whole strength and mind to a life-long movement to rid India of repression and every kind of misery.

Usually rebellion does not resolve pain. It only adds bitterness to the burden. I see this happening in so much of the rebellion that has become the feverish mood of our time. These rebellions doubtless arise because of pain, injustice, wrongs. But rebellion itself is no cure. It has no Calvary, no Easter, no Pentecost, no new age coming with glory and power. It has no Savior. Hence it cannot be redemptive. It turns out to be another form of pain itself. It amounts to little more than one pain trying to treat and heal another.

If only rebels could see that God is the Supreme Rebel (if one might put it that way). God has risen in opposition to all that has deformed his creation. He has taken all the ills and wrongs and pains of the world into himself to take them away. "In all our afflictions he was afflicted." Our Lord Jesus has personally broken the tyranny of Satan and death and his cross has become the fountain of healing waters where God makes men and nature completely whole.

God's Answer

God's answer to all of the failings, flaws, evils, and pains of this decaying, perishing old creation is the coming of a new creation. He will not put the new wine of the resurrection life into the old wineskins of the first creation, for the wineskins will burst. But he will put the new life into the new wineskin of a new creation.

And the bringer of this new creation, of this healing and restoration, is Jesus the Lord of life, who died and rose from death, who ascended to the heavens and gave his Spirit to men, and who will come again in power and great glory. To him be all praise and adoration forever. Amen!

3

Pain in Biblical Perspective

It is helpful to see pain, suffering, evil, and all their related troubles in a wide perspective. Let me explain.

Health and well-being are derivatives from the first creation. A high standard of wholeness was established by God which enabled our first parents to live and walk fully and freely in the will and purpose of God on earth. There was no evil in sight. There was never a pain, no sorrow, no suffering, no impairment such as comes through disease, accident, or old age, and no death. The issue of life was joy. No limitations of any kind robbed our first parents of the joy of life in body, mind, or spirit. Such health was not for its own sake, but it was simply God's image in his created children and it fitted them to dwell on the earth, their homeland, and to serve God with a full measure of devotion, with delight and peace, with love and adoration, world without end.

This is the way it was at the beginning, at the first creation. Now leap in thought to the end of the book, across the ages of time to the end of the world and to the fullness of the new creation. There the same full health and wholeness will again be realized in the final resurrection, in the new earth, in the Paradise restored. Again man will be in his blissful homeland, free of tears, pain, evil, and death. And God will be all in all.

Meanwhile, between the first creation's beginning and the triumph of the new creation, this wholeness and health has been disrupted, due to sin. Pain and tragedy come from brokenness, brokenness with God. It all flows from the fall of Adam and Eve as a river of pain and suffering, pouring out its bitter waters of sorrow and corruption on all people and the world. And the end of it all is death.

Now for all of us who live in this interim period between the two great creations there come three significant experiences: of the goodness in nature, of pain, and of a foretaste of the resurrection.

Goodness in Nature

There is first the experience of goodness in nature, in the world, and in life, the goodness that God built into the first creation. Not all of this perished in the judgment and in the curse of the Fall. Indeed, much of it survived on through the judgment of the Flood as well as the other judgments that have come again and again.

The earth is fruitful, beautiful, rich in wonder and resources. It awakens mankind to poetry and song, to exploration and conquest, to labor and industry. It gives to people wealth and pleasure, a home, and countless comforts. This is all the work of God and the gift of God. We did not make it.

We cannot take liberties with it for it is not ours.

There is fidelity in nature—in days and nights, seasons, and harvests—and in the laws by which the whole is held together in marvelous order. Nature is basically joy, God's joy. The Psalmist could see this and could speak of the trees clapping their hands and the stars singing their praises to God. This is the basic stuff of nature though now this is punctuated with storms, droughts, floods, disasters, and many griefs.

So we live in God's good world where he has everywhere left visible signs of his presence and power. "Ever since the creation of the world his invisible nature, namely his eternal power and deity, has been clearly perceived in the things that have been made" (Romans 1:20). His word to men is still to tame and to master the earth, to farm it, care for it, and use it to God's glory. This leaves us scope and room to work and to live for God in our lifetime in any part of the world —on land or sea or in the air—and to turn all of our activities on the earth into a service for him.

The Experience of Pain

But pain enters into our world and our lives and makes us pause. It rings a sharp warning. This world is a flawed world. It is under judgment. It is cursed. It is perishing. It is doomed. It is so thoroughly infected with the virus of sin that the only final cure for it is to be plucked up and thrown into the fire (like the raspberries in my garden which had a virus disease for which there is no cure but the bonfire).

Tornadoes cut careless swaths of destruction across farms and towns. Floods wash houses and lands away. Earthquakes toss people and their belongings around like sand and pebbles. Snakes and beasts and bugs bring fear because of the damage they do. The air overhead turns to smog and the rivers carry our pollution to the sea. Cancer, heart attacks, blindness, and blight attack young and old like robbers that strike in the night.

Pain in the body is incipient death. It is death's hand claiming us. Our bodies are of this first creation; they are of the earth; they are earthy. They perish and return to the dust. Pain is the signal, the foretaste of death. It may be only a warning signal now, but one day it will be the last call and we will have to surrender the body to the earth out of which it came, to lie there until the old creation is finally destroyed in flaming judgment.

Foretaste of the Resurrection

With the resurrection of Christ there began the new creation. Jesus rose as the second Adam, father of a new, reborn race. He ascended to rule at the throne of God to work out the agenda of the new creation. There will be a new heaven and a new earth, for the first heaven and the first earth will pass away (Revelation 21:1). The book of Revelation runs to fantastic ecstasy in describing the unspeakable glories of this new realm. The first-fruits of it have already appeared. The fullness is yet to come. It is waiting for the hour of its destiny. And it will not have long to wait for the time is close at hand.

Though it is coming, it has already come. But it is hidden from the eyes of the world. Jesus brought it. The Holy Spirit now imparts it to us by a new birth and gives to us a foretaste of the resurrection and of the new creation. Some of these previews dwell in the inner spirit of people. Some are to be seen in the gifts which the Spirit gives for our service for God. Some touches of the endless life are also given in the body, as when the Holy Spirit brings divine healing for a time. That, I think, is some of the meaning of Romans 8:11: "For if the Spirit of him who raised Jesus from the dead dwells in you, he who raised Christ Jesus from the dead will give life to your mortal bodies also through his Spirit which dwells in you."

Growth in Understanding

When I see pain and healing in perspective, I gain understanding.

- I understand that when I am reasonably well and free of illness, I know that I am enjoying the good provision of God in the first and the old creation of which I am still very much a part. And I thank God for this. At the same time I know that this is only temporary, and that at any moment I may be stricken with pain and may be brought down to death.

- I understand that when I get sick, my pains are telling me that I am mortal, that I am really dying, for my body will soon be back in the dust of this perishing creation. I accept this and make ready to lay down my body and surrender it to the earth any time, as it may please God. While I walk on this earth, I walk in the body that was made for this creation. When at last I walk on the new earth I will have a new body that will be given to me by God for that new realm.

- I understand that when the Spirit gives me foretastes of the new creation, whether by his witness of sonship, his gifts for service, his healing for my bodily pains, or his strength for life's duties, then I sing Hallelujah, for I know and believe that we shall soon be changed. "For this perishable nature must put on the imperishable, and this mortal nature must put on immortality. . . . Then shall come to pass the saying that is written: 'Death is swallowed up in victory.'"

Therefore, whether in good health, in poor health, or in Spirit-given healing, the word applies: "My beloved brethren, be steadfast, immovable, always abounding in the work of the Lord, knowing that in the Lord your labor is not in vain" (1 Corinthians 15:58).

4

The Blessings of Pain

Before I am ready to part company with pain I must pause a while to take a look at some of the amazing and astonishing transformations that come with pain as seen in the New Testament.

It looked like a judgment, now it is a mercy. It was a prison, now it is an open door. It was a dark enigma, now it works cleansing, purpose, and glory. The agonized *Why?* that throbs pathetically and insistently in the heart is silenced. Faith sees through tears, pain, and evil, and grasps the wounded hand of Jesus who has overcome darkness and all it brings, and faith sits with Jesus on his throne to wait until every enemy has been put under his feet (Ephesians 2:6).

Ages before the resurrection of Jesus, David had seen enough light to write the immortal words of comfort in Psalm 23: "Even though I walk through the valley of the shadow of death, I will fear no evil; for thou art with me."

Then the New Testament looked straight into the prison of pain and shouted a joyous Hallelujah!

- Count it all joy, my brethren, when you meet various trials (James 1:2).

- Do not be surprised at the fiery ordeal which comes upon you to prove you, as though something strange were happening to you. But rejoice insofar as you share Christ's sufferings (1 Peter 4:12-13).

- Now I rejoice in my sufferings for your sake, and in my flesh I complete what is lacking in Christ's afflictions for the sake of his body, that is, the church (Colossians 1:24).

- . . . heirs of God and fellow heirs with

Christ, provided we suffer with him in order that we may also be glorified with him (Romans 8:17).

Now what is there in the prison of pain to shout about? Certainly pain itself brings no glory.

But some secret discovery by the early Christians in this prison of suffering made them even court pain that they might get to the glory that was mysteriously associated with it.

If we ask petulantly or angrily, "Why has this happened to me?" there is no answer, for the question is locked up in *me*.

I have read that a father whose son was killed in the Viet Nam war demanded to know: "Where was God when my son was killed?" His old pastor answered kindly, "Just where he was when his own Son was killed at Calvary." The pastor turned the eyes of the distressed father to Jesus on the Cross. What happened at Golgotha transformed pain and suffering, sorrow and deviltry into a triumph.

It was a man like ourselves, and a man
with guilty blood on his hands, a man who
had to tear life out by the roots to get rid
of his pride of rank and mind, who said:
"For the sake of Christ, then, I am content
with weaknesses, insults, hardships, persecutions, and calamities; for when I am weak,
then I am strong" (2 Corinthians 12:10).
For the power of Christ is made perfect in
weakness.

Paul's word is rooted in Christ, crucified
and risen. And for Christ's sake Paul chose
and deliberately suffered the loss of all that
he cherished and clung to before he met
Christ. He suffered this loss so that "I may
gain Christ and be found in him . . . that I
may know him and the power of his resurrection, and may share his sufferings, becoming like him in his death, that if possible
I may attain the resurrection from the dead"
(Philippians 3:7-11).

What strange language! In some mysterious way pain is the route that leads to the
deepest possible knowledge and fellowship
with Christ.

All of this suggests that pain, suffering, and whatever mauling we may get from the evils of this world put us in the way of great blessing if we meet them in Christ and in his resurrection power. They then are helpers to us, servants if you like. They crowd us to Christ. But how is it possible that pain can do us any such good? Let me suggest the following:

The Way of Cleansing

Pain may put us in the way of cleansing. Many people look to God with lifelong thankfulness for an illness or an affliction or loss that somehow brought them to Christ for a deeper cleansing.

Alan Redpath, who has served as pastor in some of the largest congregations in the world, was stricken for many months with an almost fatal illness. Then after healing and restoration, he wrote: "How I thanked God for calling me aside for stillness, and how I praised him for suffering. 'It is a good thing for me that I have been afflicted' (Psalm

119:71). As I look back on it all, I would
not have missed it for anything the world
could give me. If the Lord had healed me
dramatically and instantly, what blessing I
would have missed."

And then Mr. Redpath went on to speak
of the deep cleansing he experienced as the
Lord came to him in pain. For the first time
in many months he sensed that the Lord
drew very near to him to speak to him about
his own needs, his emptiness, his sinful flesh,
his pride, his busyness with secondary things.
"The Lord showed me that I was putting
work before worship," he said. "I had become much more concerned about the
knowledge of truth than the knowledge of
God."

I will never forget the day when several
of us met at the bedside of one of God's very
able servants, a dear brother and faithful
evangelist. He lay dying. For weeks his illness had brought him down to death by slow
steps and every remedy had failed. He called
us to come to him. With feeble and broken
voice he wept out a confession of one par-

ticular trouble that had been eating like acid in his conscience and heart. We then talked together about God's merciful forgiveness and the peace of God fell on him like a gentle rain. With great relief he sank back on his pillows and prayed, "Now let your servant depart in peace, O Lord!"

But we said, "No, Lord, not so! We need him. Spare him to us!" We poured oil on him in the name of the Lord and laid our hands on him as we prayed. And in the weeks that followed he regained his strength and health and preached for fifteen more years before he died.

James says that the prayer of faith will save the sick man and the Lord will raise him up. "And if he has committed sins, they will be forgiven." Our brother's illness drew him into a deeper cleansing from sins than he had ever before experienced, all because he met his pains at the cross.

To Illuminate Our Calling

Pain can help to illuminate our calling. "He who says he abides in him ought to walk in the same way in which he walked" (1 John 2:6). At no point does the life of Jesus show up better in a disciple and follower than at the point of pain.

This is what Paul means when he says, "We are afflicted in every way . . . always carrying in the body the death of Jesus, so that the life of Jesus may also be manifested in our bodies. For while we live we are always being given up to death for Jesus' sake, so that the life of Jesus may be manifested in our mortal flesh" (2 Corinthians 4:8-11).

This throws a remarkable light on our calling, namely, to display the life of the Son of God in our bodies. And his life of resurrection, blessing, and power shows up never more clearly than in the place of pain, if we meet it at the cross.

Hudson Taylor sat with a number of new missionaries in a Chinese tea shop. After each had been served a bowl of tea, Mr. Taylor suddenly struck the table with his fist and of course the tea went spilling out of the bowls all over the table.

"In China," said Mr. Taylor, "you will receive many blows of all kinds, and then what is in you will spill out. If Christ is your life, then the life of Jesus will be manifested in your bodies whenever you are struck."

Pain may thus help us to realize our calling, which is to walk as Jesus walked and to have the life of Jesus spill out of us every time we are stricken or bruised by pain.

A Corrective for Distorted Vision

Pain is often a corrective for distorted vision. Our eyes get out of focus. Big things grow dim and hazy. Little things loom up as big, important, and urgent. We get up our blood pressure over them and we bug everyone around us with our fussiness. Then comes pain.

For this slight, momentary affliction is preparing for us an eternal weight of glory beyond all comparison, because we look not to the things that are seen but to the things that are unseen; for the things that are seen are transient, but the things that are unseen are eternal (2 Corinthians 4:17-18).

When we take afflictions to the cross we get to see things in perspective and in proportion again. Pain can thus be a corrective to our eyes.

Pain Helps Us Think of Others

Pain—when we meet it at the cross—helps us to think of others and to hold out a redemptive hand to them (rather than to judge, criticize, and condemn them).

Watch Jesus in his last agonizing hours at Calvary, bleeding and suffering, with nasty flies buzzing around his wounds, and with the heartless mob looking on.

First—he arranged to have his mother stay with John.

Next—he opened the gates of Paradise to an undeserving thief.

Then—for all his wicked foes he prayed, "Father, forgive them."

Here in pain and death his love, patience, mercy, and heart for others reached out freely to the needs of those around him.

And so too, Paul writes about learning through sufferings how to comfort others with the comfort that came to us in pain, comforts we have found at the cross of Jesus.

Pain Affects Worship

When we take our pains to the cross we will worship differently. It is one thing to sing, "I surrender all," in a modern church with all of the delightful atmosphere of quietness, fellowship, good feeling, full offering envelope, and unbroken health. It is quite another thing to sit on an ash heap, with everything lost (family, houses, herds, reputation), with broken health and running sores, with wife and friends heaping scorn on one, and there say simply—"The Lord gave, and the Lord has taken away; blessed be the name of the Lord" (Job 1:21).

We often sing, "Now thank we all our God," but few remember that this was written and sung in the midst of a destroying plague!

It was in the desolation, poverty, and bondage of the slave plantations of the deep South that the moving song of worship rose to the throne of God: "Nobody knows the trouble I've seen. Nobody knows but Jesus. Glory, Hallelujah!" This is the way the heart in pain sings and worships at the foot of the cross.

Pain Moves People to Pray

When pain comes people are moved to pray. The greatest outpouring of prayer in the Bible or anywhere else is the Psalter. "Out of the depths I cry to thee, O Lord" (Psalm 130:1). And most of this great collection of poems is a cry to God out of all kinds of pains and troubles.

Not only do people pray for themselves when pain comes, but the pains of others also move them to pray. Paul called to others to pray for him, and he more than once acknowledged the benefits that came to him because others prayed for him (as in Philippians 1:19).

Alan Redpath says: "Most comforting to me in this experience were the letters, cablegrams, and telephone calls which came to our home, assuring me of the prayers of God's people. . . . The love, thoughts, and prayers of hundreds of Christian people throughout the world were a tremendous encouragement."

5

What Can I Do About Pain?

And now there remains only one more word. What, after all is said and done, am I to do about pain? What shall I do about the pains that come to me and about the pains that I see coming to people all around me? I am still speaking of pain in its widest sense to include all the ills that have come to the world and to mankind because of our brokenness from God. If I am to come to terms with this I must be personal, simple, and direct.

I Will Accept Pain

For one thing, I will accept pain. Hear the apostle Paul say: "For the sake of Christ, then, I am content with weaknesses, insults, hardships, persecutions and calamities." That is the language of acceptance. Let me explain.

I will accept as real and actual all the pains of life, those that touch me, those that hurt other people, and those that I see in the creation around me. They are real. They are actual. They are true. They are there and they hurt. I will be honest with them and will deal with them as realistically as I can.

Some people argue that the world is becoming better, more healthy, more paradisiacal. This is the hollow optimism shared by communism, humanism, positive science, and the dream of the great American society. But broad freeways, supersonic planes, automatic washers, atomic energy, miracle computers, and medicare for everybody do not mean that the cancerous pains of the old creation are being cured. They are still malignant and they break out in new troubles, if not in leprosy and malaria, then in mental disorders, moral decay, and in social strife. For the old creation is rotting away. It is dy-

ing. The pains and the sufferings we see in
ourselves and in others are but personal, im-
mediate, and intimate tastes of the universal
malady. The basis of life under the curse of
sin is tragic. It has no cure in and of itself.
Its course is fatal. Its end is despair. For this
world with all its ills is reserved for a final
termination "in flaming fire . . . when the
earth and the works upon it shall be burned
up" (2 Thessalonians 1:8 and 2 Peter 3:10).
I accept the realism of this.

There is sorrow in all of this too and this
is no less real. I will accept the sorrows. I
will not be ashamed to weep and to sorrow,
to groan and to suffer at the sight and the
touch of pains. My Savior cried on the cross,
"I thirst!" and I will be honest too about the
pains I feel.

Others understand if I weep when pains
come to me personally. We expect this. But
Jesus expects me to sorrow when others sorrow, to weep when others weep, to remember those who are in bonds as being bound
with them. Jesus himself did this when he
stood at the tomb of Lazarus. With all our

afflictions he was afflicted. He took our infirmities and bore our sicknesses. And "Christ also suffered for you, leaving you an example that you should follow in his steps" (1 Peter 2:21).

There is also a suffering in nature, a groaning under its pains. And I want to be able to groan with the earth in its "travails" when fires destroy the forests, when rivers are polluted by filth, or when the cities are smothered in choking smog.

Pain is real, actual, hurtful, harsh, cruel, destructive. This cannot be evaded or somehow softened by perfume, roses, soft music, as when the undertaker gave me a handful of rose petals to scatter on the top of a casket at the grave in place of dirt, as I came to pronounce the fateful words of God: "You are dust, and to dust you shall return!" God did not mute the harshness of those awful words. He did not substitute roses for dirt and dust. Nor will I. It is too terribly real, and I will accept this as God has made it to be. This alone is true realism and honesty with things as they are.

I will accept pain as belonging rightfully to this world in which I dwell. It is not something accidental. It did not sneak in under the fence somehow. It is not here on a forged passport. It is not some kind of a mistake, or an unfortunate mutation. Pain is in this world because it has a right to be here. It can strike F.D.R. with polio, it can sink the Titanic, it can blast Hiroshima with a great burst of hell-fire, it can pour heresy into the church, it can behead the saints. It has a command and an authority to roam the earth until the last day of the world.

The Bible links natural and culpable evil. Natural evil and pain are always the visible sign of God's *No!* which he pronounced on creation and on man because of the sinful alienation of man from God. Ever since the gate to the garden was shut and the angel of the Lord was placed there to guard it with a flaming two-edged sword—ever since that day the earth has been filled with violence and thistles, pain and disorder, decay and despair. The twisted life of man is a tragic modification of God's intention and purpose.

In one sense this is only temporary, for it will not continue thus forever. It will end in fire. In another sense this is permanent, for its nature will never improve. Healing of any kind, improvement of any sort will be incomplete, momentary. It will alleviate suffering for a brief while, no more. It points to the great coming day when in God's new creation sorrow, tears, sickness, evil, and death will be at an end. But for as long as the earth lasts it will continue in pain. This will be its native element. *God has decided it shall be so.* This is how he is handling the situation. *Therefore it is right that it be this way.* And therefore I accept pain as the legitimate right and the true heritage of a cursed and stricken world.

And God said to Adam: "Because you have disobeyed, cursed is the ground because of you; in toil you shall eat of it all the days of your life; thorns and thistles it shall bring forth to you. In the sweat of your face you shall eat bread till you return to the ground, for out of it you were taken; you are dust, and to dust you shall return" (Genesis 3:17-19).

Now, if I accept pain as right for the earth I will accept it as right for me, too, since in my body I am of the dust of the earth and thus share in the actual matter and destiny of the old creation. Though we are the children of God and have been delivered with Christ out of this evil world, we are still in it and together with the rest of the world we sit in Satan's lap (1 John 5:19). The pains that come from this evil situation affect all who live in this world.

Cars crash and kill 50,000 people a year in this country, leaving many more thousands broken and crippled for months or for years. Wars damn us all to misery and loss. Sickness is in the air we breathe, in the food we eat, even in our blood stream. Demons prowl the earth to strike men as they please. The Reds murder 50 million people in the first five years of their takeover in China, Christians and non-Christians alike, and shut down all the churches and outlaw religious faith. Yesterday one of the young men of our congregation is drowned in the river. Today a neighbor is robbed and beaten in his store. Tomorrow I may have a heart attack, or be given surgery for cancer, and never walk again.

We are all partners (with Chinese and Africans, with Hindus and communists, with rich and poor) in the earth's bankruptcy. We are all stockholders in a vast and ruinous failure. The proof of this is death. Nobody escapes death. Nobody goes to his own funeral and then comes home again. Nobody! Ever! And so I will accept this, not only as right for the world, but as right for me too, since I too am dust. This is God's doing, his judgment, and I accept it as such.

I will accept pain for Jesus' sake. By this I mean that no matter what pains come to me I will accept as coming from the hand of God.

Jesus did this. Satan fixed the bitter cup of his suffering and served it to him by brutal force. Jesus said that he could call down 12 legions of angels to unarm his foes, but he did not do it. Instead he took the cup to his

Father and prayed: "If it be possible, let this cup pass from me. Nevertheless, not my will but thine be done." And the Father did not remove the cup from him. The Father did not spare him. So Jesus took the cup from the Father's hand and drank it to its dregs! When the mercenary soldiers came to capture him in the garden, he "allowed himself" (literally) to them.

Job did this. All was lost, all but his heartbeat. He touched absolute bottom. Satan beat him down to within an inch of his life. His friends condemned him. His wife urged him to curse God and die. But as Job listened to all of this, as he saw the desolation all around him, as he scraped the puss from his stinking sores with a broken bit of pottery, he did not curse his bad luck. He did not blame Satan for what had happened. He did not complain to God. Instead he saw the hand of God in it all and he said firmly: "The Lord gave, and the Lord has taken away; blessed be the name of the Lord."

David did this. Absalom, David's favorite son, was a traitor to his father. He raised an army of rebels and marched against Jerusalem to throw his father off the throne. David was unsuspecting, unprepared, and left the city. In sorrow, suffering, and humiliation David walked out of the city with his family and certain followers and leaders who were faithful to him. From across a ravine a man named Shimei shouted taunts and curses at David and threw dust and stones in derision at him. David's general who walked beside him growled to David in anger, "Let me go over and strike off that dog's head." But David forbade him, saying, "No, do him no harm, for the Lord has said to Shimei, 'Curse David!'" Thus David took the curses of a miserable traitor as coming from the mouth of God!

Madame Guyon looked upon her cell in the French prison as a cage, God's cage, and she saw herself as God's canary, placed there by the Lord to sing for his delight. So she wrote her sweetest songs and sang her most moving melodies in France's great prisons, bound there for the sake of her faith in Jesus, and praised God for putting her there in his cage to sing for him.

The English martyr, condemned for his evangelical faith under the reign of Bloody Mary, climbed the scaffold and cried aloud: "Thanked be God! These be God's front steps and I am even now at home!"

Mr. Anderson was for many years a helpless invalid in Veterans' Hospital in Minneapolis. Many of us who went to visit him came away with our hearts lifted to the throne of God. In the last days of his life he was twisted into painful contortions by arthritis. He could hardly move. But his eyes sparkled with a deep knowledge and glory as he spoke of the goodness of God to him. To him the Vets' Hospital was God's house. His bed was God's footstool. His arthritis was a robe that God had given him to wear (Jesus wore it too, he once said with a wink, for Jesus took our infirmities and *bore*—or rather *wore* our sicknesses.) The nurses were angels who cared for him. He never complained, only praised God and blessed everybody. In this way he took each day as a gift from

God's hand and turned it into a ministry and service of praise and worship of praise and worship to God.

All of this demonstrates an accepting faith —a faith that welcomes pains, ills, necessities, adversities for Christ's sake, seeing God's loving hand in all that happens, thus giving thanks always in everything because this is the will of God for you (Ephesians 5:20 and Colossians 3:17). This attitude of acceptance calls to me. I will follow.

Faith involves more than acceptance— even joyful, thankful acceptance (free and wonderful as that can be!). St. Paul takes pleasure in weaknesses and in calamities, and he all the more gladly boasts in weaknesses, not just for Christ's sake, but also because Christ's power is made perfect in weakness. He said that he embraced pains so that the power of Christ might rest upon him.

We call to God for healing, for deliverance because we have the strong notion that God's great glory and power are at their best and displayed most effectively in health, strength, and in everything going good and well. Paul reverses this notion and claims to see God's power best displayed and working most effectively in weakness, in calamity, in necessities—even in pain!

Somehow in the grasp of faith the fiery darts of the evil one are not just shielded off. They are used to turn loose the saving power of God (as in the Philippi jail by Paul and Silas). Tragedies are forged into triumphs. The valley of weeping becomes an oasis with flowing springs. Faith has moved from submission, from contentment, from acceptance, to adventure and to conquest. The attack of Goliath against a teenager with nothing but a sling is turned into a victory that routs the whole Philistine army. David not only accepted the attack, he used it!

Our Lord Jesus is the supreme example of this. Born in lowliness, grown up in obscurity, going about as an itinerant teacher and preacher, supported by the little gifts and donations mainly from women (Luke 8:3), rejected, hated, put to death, buried in another man's grave. But he used all this. He deliberately took this route. Though he was rich, he became poor purposefully that we *through his poverty* might become rich.

I confess that this prospect draws my heart with a great attraction. The greatest triumph of Christian confidence is reached not by leapfrogging over pain and death to live in the imagery of a world of miraculous healings and deliverances now, and then of perfection beyond the grave, but by taking death in the midst of daily life and making it the servant of redemption.

Death is swallowed up. That sounds like a clue. The believer is someone who has taken death into his system and turned it into a way of life. Pain and death are not something that come and happen to us, but rather they are something we do.

"I die daily," said Paul. "We who live are continually being delivered up to death for Jesus' sake . . . so death works in us." "For I think that God has exhibited us apostles as last of all, like men sentenced to death." "Whatever gain I had, I counted as loss for the sake of Christ. For his sake I have suffered the loss of all things . . . that I may share in his sufferings, becoming like him in his death."

All of this is strange language but it marks out a pattern, a road to be followed, a way of life to be lived. It does two things for the Christian.

1. *A Christian makes a practice of daily dying to this old world.* The final death of the body will then be the final loss to which all the other daily deaths lead. He does most of his essential dying in advance of death. This should not be something surprising, for we were baptized into a way of death and life. Not only were we sacramentally identified in the dying and rising of Jesus, but we were committed to a continual repetition of the pattern of the grain of wheat that falls into the ground and dies in order to bear fruit. The dying and rising of Jesus is the authentic pattern of life with God, in him and in us too.

2. *The cross of Jesus demonstrated how God uses pain, loss, evil, and death to bring about good.* He took the fiercest attack of Sa-

tan and turned it into the instrument of salvation for the world.

Similarly, God has taken some of the worst afflictions that have come into the lives of his people and has turned these into routes of blessing for families, tribes, and nations. In this way many believers have been allowed to "complete what is lacking in Christ's afflictions for the sake of his body" (Colossians 1:24).

Thus many Christians have risen up in weakness, in loss, in affliction, to walk and work and minister in the power of Christ to an extent and in a measure they never dreamed possible.

"When I am weak, *then* I am strong," said the Apostle Paul, for the "power of Christ is made perfect in weakness."

Mr. and Mrs. Lee saw this when their house and family were swept away in a monsoon storm in the Himalayas. And out of this tragic loss they turned to rescue hundreds and thousands of Hindu girls in Calcutta.

Daniel T. Niles came home and wept on the night that the Ceylon government took over all the Christian schools. The church and missions provided 90 percent of the schools in Ceylon. "This is the end of Christianity in Ceylon," he moaned and mourned the great loss. But somehow the striking words of the apostle stole into his mind— "made perfect in weakness . . . when I am weak, then I am strong." When the light of this flooded his mind he rose up with a new joy and welcomed the loss as being the greatest opportunity that there could be for the power of Christ now to do its work in the weakness of the church!

So much for acceptance. The first thing I will do with pain then is to accept it.

I Will Tackle Pain

Now the second thing I will do with pain is to tackle it, assail it, lay my hands on it and remove it if at all possible. Jesus did this all through his public ministry. Even as he surrendered himself to the cruel tortures of his tormentors he asked for a moment to put an ear back on a man's head after Peter had slashed it off with a sword. And he sent his disciples out into the countryside with the charge: "Heal the sick, raise the dead, cleanse lepers, cast out demons. You received without paying, give without pay" (Matthew 10:8).

Therefore I will use the tools and means that God has given us in this old creation for keeping pains in check and for cultivating health, wholeness, and well-being. There are many good measures for working at this. There are the physical benefits of good food, rest and exercise; the help of herbs, medicines, surgery, and many kinds of therapy; the mysterious power to heal that there is in the touch of some specially endowed people; the improvement that can come by change in climate, occupation, or habitation; the curative power of good and wholesome attitudes as emphasized so strongly by men like E. Stanley Jones.

For the preservation and welfare of the whole human family we do the best we can with education, government, industry, commerce, the arts, communications, and much more.

And for the conservation and cultivation of the resources and fruits of the earth we now have the amazing tools of science, exploration, and control, plus the human talents of three and a half billion people who are scattered everywhere in the world.

I know that what I can do about using these tools is very little and I weep to think of what a great job there is to do. But even a few people working hard at this can keep the weeds from covering the whole ground. These are the means God has given us to cultivate the earth and to make the very best of human life on it. He blesses these tools and supports those who employ them for the good and benefit of people. Therefore I am for them. I will support them and I will use them all I can—from the medicine cabinet in the bathroom to the more sophisticated and complex instruments and institutions that have enriched our lives by all the good that they have done.

But there are spiritual tools as well. These

are the instruments of the New Creation. They are hidden to all but to the eyes of faith. And they too are powerful to tear down all that is opposed to God and to bring in the light, the power, the life, and the health of God's kingdom among men.

There is the Bible, by which men may escape from the corruptions that are in the world because of lust and may become partakers of the divine nature. There is prayer and faith, by which men have carried out the greatest exploits for good through the power of God (Hebrews 11). There is the cleansing, healing, strengthening fellowship of the church, the family of God. There are the sacraments, the gifts of the Holy Spirit, and the testimony and witness of believing Christian people.

Sometimes the powers of the resurrection life burst out in rivers of spiritual revival, as in the days of the Wesleys in England, through which England was saved from the kind of blood-bath that came to France in its terrifying revolution.

Sometimes, the power of God comes in

bodily healing, in physical renewal, in special skills and abilities, spiritual gifts, and heightened talents.

Sometimes the glories of the resurrection life shine in suffering, as happened on the face of Stephen while he was being stoned to death outside the city.

Much more often, and far less dramatically, the presence, power, and life of Jesus are shown in his people as they marry in his name, rear their children in his name, attend the meetings of the congregation in quiet faith, support the work of God's kingdom with sacrifice and faithfulness, hold to the truth always in speech and in work, show patience, love, and understanding for others, keep their tongues from anger, meanness, and gossip, and give thanks unfailingly to God for all things and at all times because this is the will of God for them. They are, more than anybody else, the salt of the earth and the light of the world. The health and life of the New Age in them (God working in them) helps to keep the world from going completely to pot before its final end comes.

The Mystery of Pain

It is from my Lord Jesus Christ (particularly at the cross) that I first learn to accept pain. And then I also learn from him to use all the tools I can to heal hurts, remove pain, alleviate sufferings, and lift the burdens of sorrow and woe wherever they are found.

You may say this is contradictory. I say it is a paradox, for paradox is not an untruth or a deception. Both of its seemingly contradictory terms are verified in Christ Jesus, and in the daily life of those in whom God dwells and in whom he works "both to will and to do his good pleasure."

This is a great part of the mystery surrounding pain!

About the Author

The doctor looked Paul Lindell straight in the eye and said, "I'm going to give it to you straight. You have cancer." This is how Paul learned that he had a terminal illness. The news came to him on the birthday of his only son, March 17, 1969. On Friday, March 1, 1974 his promotion came. Out of the five years of pain, question, thought, and an intimate relationship with Jesus Christ and his family, came Paul's personal expression of faith, *The Mystery of Pain.*

What kind of man was Paul Lindell? Who was he and what did he do? The record of his wrestling with the ultimate issues of life indicates that he was no ordinary man.

Paul J. Lindell, eldest of three sons, was born August 13, 1915 to godly missionary parents, Rev. and Mrs. Johan J. Lindell, on the mountains of Kikungshan, Honan, China. His brother Jonathan is a missionary to Nepal and his brother David is a missionary to South India. Schooled in China until ready for college, Paul attended Gustavus Adolphus College in St. Peter, Minnesota three years, and the University of Minnesota one year. He then studied one year each at Augsburg Seminary, Minneapolis, and Augustana Seminary, Rock Island, Illinois. Following one year of congregational internship at Calvary Lutheran Church, Minneapolis, 1939-1940, Paul married Margaret Sovik, who also had grown up in China, on August 23, 1940. Together they joined the home staff of the World Mission Prayer League, a Lutheran missionary fellowship. In this assignment they found their Christian calling and life work.

When I was a teenager I knew Paul as a dynamic missionary leader. I first met him at Christmas, 1941, when I traveled with his younger brother, David, to Minneapolis. As we entered Paul and Margaret's home a giant banner greeted us. It showed a conquistador with raised sword emphasizing this phrase from the book of Hebrews, "Be not sluggish but imitators of those who through faith and patience inherit the promises." I met not only a young man of twenty-six but a way of life. His life was a compelling example of radical discipleship to Jesus Christ expressing itself in total missionary obedience. Paul expressed this missionary obedience in his leadership of the World Mission Prayer League. He served as its General Director for 33 years.

The World Mission Prayer League is a fellowship of about 120 missionaries serving in Afghanistan, Bolivia, Ecuador, India, Mexico, Zaire, Nepal, Bangladesh, and Pakistan. They express their commitment to Jesus Christ in lives of Christian service, witness, and presence. This missionary fellowship is in the tradition of such groups as Hudson Taylor's China Inland Mission in that it does not guarantee financial support but rather pledges itself to prayer and faith on behalf of the missionary family and forwards such resources that come its way. Paul's example of dependence on God is written indelibly on all who have a part in this missionary fellowship. His life was a channel of God's resources for all who knew him and worked with him.

Beginning in 1954 I developed a new and deeper understanding of Paul when I was called by the Lutheran World Federation to be a missionary to Africa. As a fellow worker in the missionary vocation I learned that Paul had a concern for the total Christian missionary outreach. He was as happy with my missionary obedience through my church as with any of his fellow workers in the World Mission Prayer League. This largeness of heart and generosity of spirit is the measure of the man. He was not parochial and exclusive, but broad and inclusive.

In 1968 my relationship with Paul took another form when I became his pastor. Paul and Margaret have been faithful members of Trinity church and have supported the work of the congregation in every way. Paul was a competent theologian, a missionary statesman, an able administrator, and an emphatic counselor. But undergirding it all he was a Christian in a local congregation of believers. To live in his company was to be affirmed and encouraged. But never was his witness more productive and effective than his living with Christ in the school of suffering.

Five years ago Paul came to our church council and in accordance with James 5:13-16 asked for a service of anointing with oil and prayer for healing. Unforgettable is the image of this servant of God, drawn in face and body as he came to his brothers in Christ in simple faith to rest his case with God.

During the next five years Paul lived in the tension between a deteriorating physical body and his growing faith. Questions were hurled at him. "Why? Why? Why?" At times he assumed the posture of Job under the gentle and loving but insistent and intimidating queries. "If you are a man of faith why are you not healed? Believe more! Confess more!" This is the furnace in which the gold of this book was refined.

In walking with Paul through many experiences and changes I was amazed at new dimensions of his faith and understanding. The last words of witness Paul wrote were these: "The daily quest of my heart before God has found its best expression in Jeremiah 17:14: 'Heal me, O Lord, and I shall be healed; save me and I shall be saved for *thou art my praise,*' and also, 'I have set the Lord always before me; I have no good apart from him. The Lord is my chosen portion and my cup. He holds my lot.' These additional words from Psalm 16 bear out the same idea and truth. So I leave my lot in God's hands and praise him for whatever this may bring to me. Healing and salvation are both equally his provision and his work. 'Therefore my heart is glad and my soul rejoices; my body also dwells secure' (Ps. 16:9). It is here that I rest and abide."

Concerning instructions for his funeral he wrote, "The scriptures which have ministered the most to me for a long time as a preparation for death have been the six verses in Psalm 23. These have been a special means of grace for living and walking through the valley of the shadow of death. I have preached on these words in public and I have moved through their majestic lanes of goodness and mercy almost constantly by day and by night in my own soul. Out of the abyss of our personal needs men have looked longingly to the heights and have cried for help. 'O God, if you wish for our love fling us a handful of stars.' God heard that cry. Heaven hungered for the love of the earth, and so his stars were flung to us in rich profusion. A cluster of these glittering stars are bunched together in Psalm 23. Here we can pick them up and thread them on strings of faith. With these we may step into today and tomorrow with courage and hope towards God and with an open hand to share our treasures."

Paul's book is a handful of stars flung out to fellow sufferers in a very real world. It comes out of a life that was disciplined in flinging itself out to the world's needs as a way of life and commends itself to us to do the same.

There are cedars of Lebanon. There are oaks of God's planting in Zion. They have been hewn and have been placed in the temple of God. Through them we have been sheltered, blessed, challenged, convicted, and cleansed. Such a tree of God's planting was Paul Lindell. He was no more and no less than a forgiven sinner, an earthen vessel, and a man of like passions; but he allowed Jesus, the Lord, to mold, dominate, and use his earthly pilgrimage.

He taught us about single-hearted and complete dedication to God's call for our life. He taught us about being renewed through using our minds to contemplate and to meditate on the claims of the kingdom of God. He showed us by walking with us into uncharted territory, unfulfilled missionary beckonings of God. He led us in simple and quiet trust that God provides resources of grace for his people and resources of common things to do God's work.

In life, in sufferings, in home-going, his steady, disciplined, daily witness always was, "I have rested my case with Jesus."

We thank God that our pilgrim work has been encouraged by one who trusted in the mystery of God's grace amid the mystery of suffering and whose single-hearted devotion could confess with that other missionary Paul, "All I want is to know Christ and experience the power of his resurrection; to share in his sufferings and to become like him in his death, in the hope that I myself will be raised from death to life."

CARL JOHANSSON